Anke Rüsbüldt

# Mud Fever

Prevention – Diagnosis – Treatment

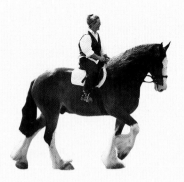

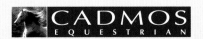

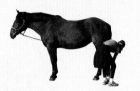

# Contents

*The Publisher advises that all of the treatments described in this book should only be undertaken in consultation with a veterinarian, and can accept no liability for their results.*

# Imprint

Copyright of original edition ©2003
Cadmos Verlag GmbH, Lüneberg.
Copyright of this edition ©2003 Cadmos Verlag.
Translated by Claire Williams
Design and typesetting: Ravenstein, Verden.
Photographs: Schmelzer, Slawik
Drawings: Susanne Retsch-Amschler
Printed by Westermann Druck, Zwickau

ISBN 3-86127-935-5

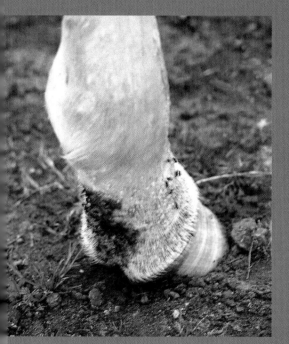

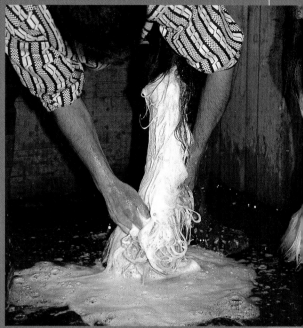

Photo titles: Here you can clearly see the affects of mud fever. (Photo H.Ende)

Treatment is more time-consuming and less pleasant than preventative action. (Photo C. Slawik)

# What is mud fever?

Mud fever is a skin infection usually affecting the back of the pastern, fetlock and the heels. The term itself is more a colloquial description than a strict medical term, and cracked heel, greasy heel, heel bug and scratches all refer to the same problem, which can also affect other areas of the body such as the upper legs and belly. There are a number of different factors w which can combine to produce the symptoms of mud fever. Similarly there are many treatments, therapies and magic potions that are recommended and used. In all cases the condition is annoying for the horse and its owner/rider, and the process of healing can be long-drawn out in the extreme. In some cases mud fever can also be extremely painful, occasionally leading to lameness and the necessity for total rest.

Medically speaking, mud fever is the term generally given to a dermatophilus infection of the lower limbs, when the skin is invaded by a bacterium called Dermatophilus congolensis. This type of infection can also be worsened by conditions such as mite infestation, fungal infections, skin damaged by abrasions and chafing, allergic dermatitis and can itself be a symptom of a more serious inner illness or a suppressed immune system.

The condition afflicts the upper layer of the skin (epidermis), but can extend through the entire skin and the under layer of the skin (hypodermis). In extreme cases secondary infection may set in affecting the lymph glands

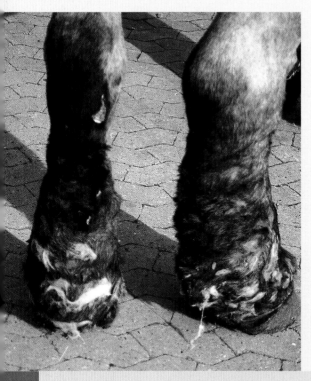

*This case has reached an almost incurable state. (Photo: H. Ende)*

hair around their fetlocks (so-called feathers), such as Clydesdales, Friesens or Irish Draughts and crosses, the problem can be difficult to recognise, and even harder to treat. It seems that horses with more feathering may be more prone to suffer from mud fever.

Mud fever also seems to be more prevalent on white legs. It can even be the case that a horse with white markings on three legs has mud fever on these, while the fourth leg remains healthy. As with nearly all skin conditions, however, Chestnuts seem more prone to it than horses of other colours.

Mud fever is not contagious. When a healthy, non-prone horse shares grazing with a horse suffering from mud fever, there is no danger of cross-infection.

*This horse is a typical candidate for mud fever: white legs, feathers and it's winter as well. Photo: C. Slawik*

and the blood, resulting in septicaemia. Similarly this can also lead to inflammation of the coronary band that can in turn affect hoof growth. When viewed in the broadest sense, as cracked heels, in advanced stages the condition can take the form of chronic, proliferative mud fever, which is only curable, if at all, by surgery. The condition is in all cases more than just a small spot of bother.

## When does it occur?

Mud fever occurs most frequently during the winter months. When it affects horses with long

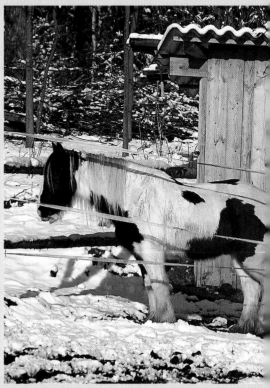

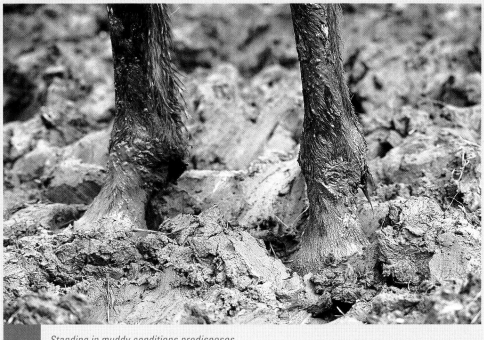

*Standing in muddy conditions predisposes horses to mud fever. (Photo: C. Slawik)*

There is a range of factors that can contribute to mud fever. It is important to remember that horses can be prone to the condition to a greater or lesser degree. It is possible that the tendency is hereditary. The condition of the animal can also play a great role. A healthy horse with a strong immune system is better able to fight off infection than one with a depressed immune system. Immunity can be weakened through general illness, bad management and care, poor feed or stress.

Advocates of natural healing and complementary medicine often assume that all skin conditions are a sign of an inner imbalance, or can be linked with a psychological problem. That may seem far-fetched, but nevertheless contented horses do appear to recover faster from infection.

Incorrect feeding can also increase the chances of mud fever occurring. In the past, brewery dray-horses often suffered from a form of craked heel which was directly related to the brewer's wash (swill), a by-product from the brewing of beer which comprised the major part of the horses' diet.

The environment in which the animal is kept is an important factor in causing disease. If the horse is kept in poor or unhygienic conditions – poorly drained pasture, a stable that is not mucked out regularly, or even bedding that may cause skin irritations – then these can all be direct causes of the condition. Irritation may be caused by medication, disinfectant, road salt or salts used to keep manege surfaces from freezing, abrasive sand or wood-chip surfaces and even straw that may prick and penetrate skin – all are potential irritants. Whether these irritants are a direct cause or whether they cause an allergic reaction may vary, but both are possible.

Once the skin is traumatised, the way is opened for bacteria and fungi. Both make their way in through small wounds and set up their own infections.

Tiny chorioptic mange mites (similar to those causing scabies in humans) can also infest the hair follicles of the lower limb around the time when coats grow out and can cause considerable skin irritation, leading to inflammation of both the pastern and fetlock areas. This condition is accompanied by an increased tendency to rub – again seen as either a direct or allergic reaction . Fungal infections can also be responsible for skin damage. Neither the mites nor the fungus mentioned here are susceptible to antibiotics, so the condition is difficult to cure.

Some horses suffer from mud fever even in the absence of any of the above causes. Others never suffer, even though all of these causes are present. It is annoying, but a fact of life and one which no one has been able to fully explain.

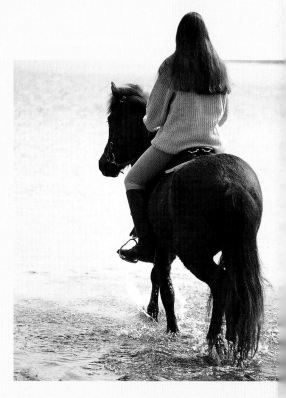
*Water alone doesn't hurt . Photo: A. Schmelzer*

## Correct management – the be all and end all

So what, in terms of horse management and care, increases the chances for mud fever? It's obvious isn't it: turning horses out in muddy conditions! That's the first thing that occurs to everyone. But it's not as simple as that.

What is true is that a misunderstanding of what comprises appropriate equine husbandry can be damaging . Horses should not be made to stand continuously in the wet. Paddocks or former pastures, which are used over the winter months are often muddy. That alone doesn't harm. Mud can only be damaging when, over time, there is less and less soil, and more and more droppings and urine are mixed in. It is also damaging when, over a continuous twenty-four hour period, it covers the bottom twenty centimetres of the horse's legs.

Of course we all want to keep our horse in the best possible conditions. This includes allowing them to spend as much time as possible outdoors with other horses. Ideally, the turnout should be relatively dry and not too deep. This, however, is not always easy to put into practice, perhaps due to personal or financial reasons, as well as a lack of time. In all cases however a horse should be kept so that it has

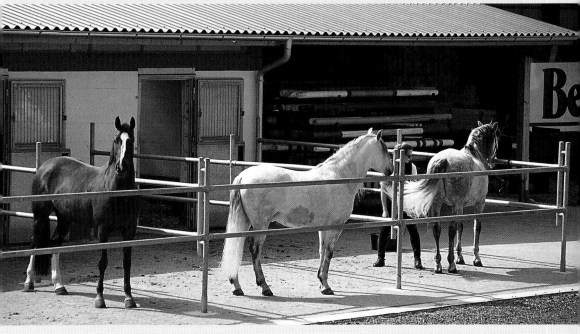

*In conditions such as these, with clean stables and paved turnout, mud fever is less likely to occur. (Photo: A. Schmelzer)*

*Mud fever can arise from damp and dirty stabling.
Photo: C. Slawik*

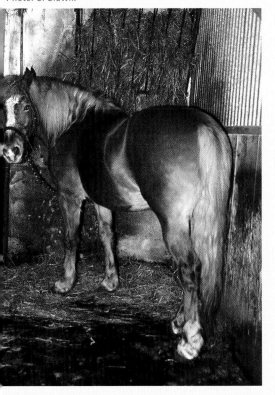

the opportunity of spending some time in a dry environment.

A field shelter that only offers the two highest-ranking horses room is no good either. Winter turnout needs to either only be used for short periods of time when attached to a stable or it needs to offer a dry retreat that all horses can use at the same time. A dry, inviting area available to all horses will also then be used by all. The feeding area, where all the horses will spend much of their time, must also be situated out of the wet. The area around drinking troughs should also be kept as clean as possible.

Turnout itself should be mucked out regularly. This involves a lot of work, but is more beneficial than you can ever imagine.

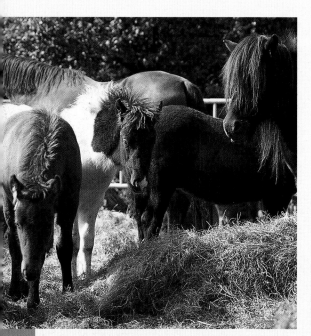

Horses spend longer around the areas where they are fed. Even though it is dry here at the moment, this form of feeding is not ideal. Photo: A. Schmelzer.

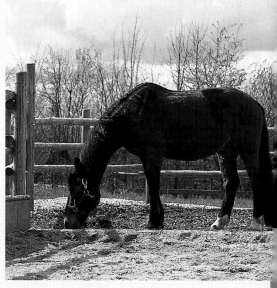

Here the surface is a mixture of sand and wood chips. Photo: C. Slawik.

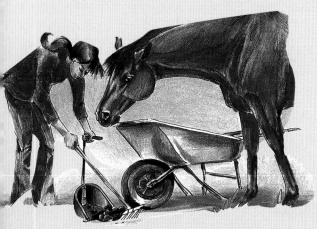

A job that's really worth doing.

It may be possible to lay drainage into a part of the turnout area, or to put down a hard surface. You can even bulldoze all the mud into one heap, that once dried creates a hill on which it will always be dry!

Sand surfaces usually don't last much more than one winter and can, when unwashed (and more expensive) river sand is used, lead to increased wear on hooves. The washed river sand combines with droppings, making them harder to remove.

Wood chips can also contain particles that are irritating for horses' legs and also mulch down within one year. Longer-lasting methods of keeping areas for turnout dry are always relatively expensive, albeit only once. They are

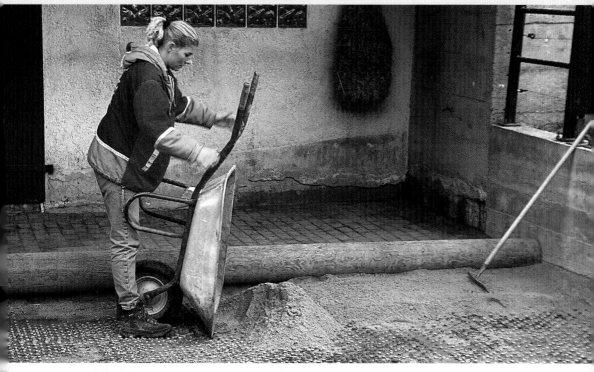

*Creating a new surface is time-consuming and expensive- but only once.
It does create good conditions which last longer. Photo: C. Slawik*

*Here you can see various solutions which create a
permanent surface. Photo: C Slawik.*

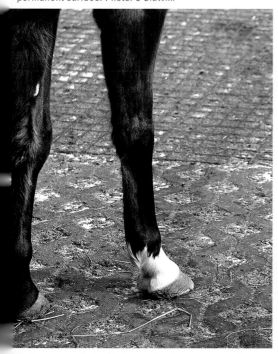

frequently also more time and work intensive, although the effort is worthwhile. Removing the surface down to a deep level and then putting down new surfaces in layers is just as suitable as a professional solution. Options are plastic grids, embedded into the ground, rubber matting and various forms of paving.

A good solution is offered by so-called "cow matting", a form of carpet over which is placed a thin layer of surface soil or similar and which ensures that water can drain away without the ground becoming waterlogged.

If horses are stabled, then the bedding should always be dry on top. Even where a deep litter system is used, the uppermost layer should be dry. Removal of droppings is also advisable, again from deep litter as well.

Any mixture of droppings and urine can, over time, irritate skin and hooves.

All types of bedding are suitable as long as it is looked after and changed often enough. There will always be horses that manage to turn their stable into a pig-sty within the space of a day. In these cases, it is easier to keep it dry with chopped straw, wood shavings or hemp, which must, of course, still be changed regularly.

In the case of a horse whose skin is already damaged in the pastern or heel area, you should be particularly careful about which chemicals are used in stables around it. As a preventative measure, commercially available ammonia powder used to reduce odours may be used.

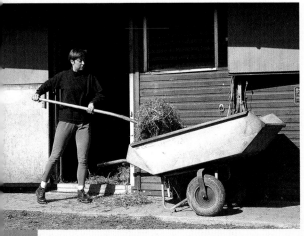

*Daily mucking out of stables is essential, otherwise your horse's skin and hooves will be needlessly irritated. Photo: A. Schmelzer*

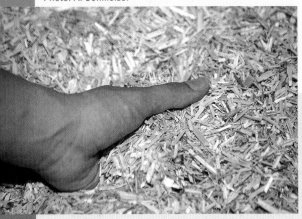

*Hemp bedding is extremely absorbent. It tends not to be eaten so unlike straw won't keep a horse occupied. Photo: A. Schmelzer*

*Normal straw can also be replaced with chopped straw. This can however lead to digestive problems when consumed in large quantities. Photo: A. Schmelzer.*

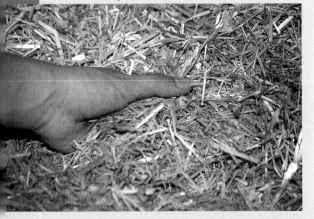

## Daily care

At the first suspicion of mud fever even possibly becoming an issue, the daily inspection and cleaning of all four legs should be automatic. And this is where the mistakes begin.

Cleaning legs daily by washing is wrong. This can be harmful and can even encourage the onset of mud fever. It is better simply to let any mud or dirt dry, and then brush it off.

Since softer body brushes usually have no real impact on the dirt a stiffer brush (such as a dandy brush) will need to be used. Be careful not to use brushes with particularly sharp or damaged bristles, however, as these can cause minute injuries that open the way for mud fever to set in.

Should you have to hose down or wash the pastern, be sure to dry off the joint thoroughly

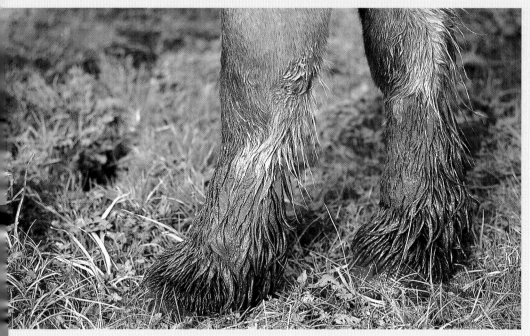

*Muddy hooves are best brushed once the mud has dried off,
as too frequent washing does more harm than good. Photo: C. Slawik*

*Dandy brushes are best suited for brushing off.
Photo: C. Slawik*

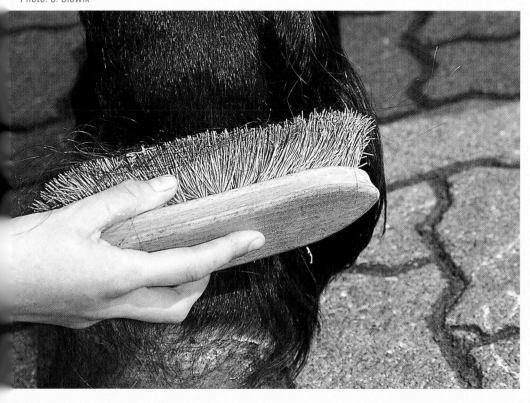

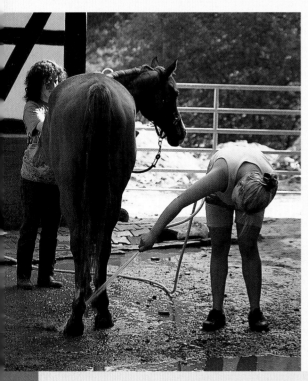

Hose down legs as little as possible.
Photo: A. Schmelzer

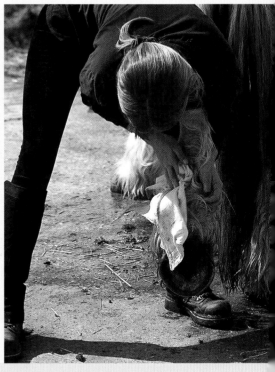

After washing, dry off the pastern gently,
not by rubbing vigorously. Photo: C. Slawik

afterwards. Use a dry, soft hand towel to gently dab away the moisture, as rubbing can irritate the skin. The towel should be regularly replaced; when it is washed, avoid using fabric conditioners as these can aggravate skin.

Feathers are sensible accessories and should not be cut off if at all possible. Only when faced with a persistent case of mud fever which may be hidden or untreatable under the long hair, should they be removed. In all other cases they are best left on. On the one hand this hair acts as a useful protection mechanism, and on the other hand it acts as a useful drainage system, channelling water down past the sensitive area around the back of the pastern- even where there is only light feathering. Regrowth

of trimmed hair and the cut hair stubble itself can prove to be an irritant that is best avoided.

Preventative application of creams and such tends as a rule to be more harmful than beneficial. Even when you think you have dried off the hair by towelling, there is still likely to be some dampness present in the hair or on the skin. Just think how your own skin feels after a long hot bath, often feeling damp even when you have dried yourself thoroughly. The best and perhaps only method of drying the legs totally is to use a hair dryer (which should be fitted with a power breaker). Most horses will tolerate it and find it far more comfortable than being towelled.

If damp skin is covered with greasy lotion, then between the two a small airtight space is

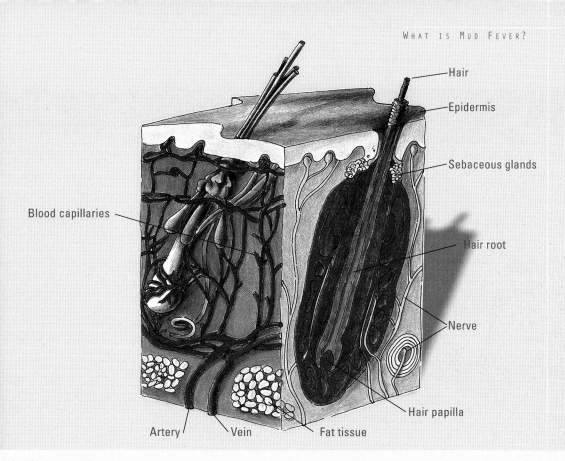

Hair

Epidermis

Sebaceous glands

Hair root

Nerve

Blood capillaries

Hair papilla

Artery

Vein

Fat tissue

*In this cross-section you can see the complex construction of skin.*

created – similar to an incubator – and it is impossible to avoid the presence of any germs there, which will be delighted at the opportunity presented! In addition, when greasy lotions are applied they are likely to pick up dirt and mud within a short space of time and this combination creates a good medium for bacteria, fungus and parasites.

As well as this, you will be blocking the pores. The layers of skin work like a protective shield against any penetrating irritations. That is how it is designed and constructed. Our aim should be to utilise the natural properties of the skin to maintain and support it; interfering with this cannot be right.

If tendon or brushing boots, over-reach boots or similar are going to be used, ensure that they are placed onto legs that are clean and dry. If not, small injuries might occur that could encourage the onset of mud fever. A few grains of sand under over-reach boots can act like sandpaper.

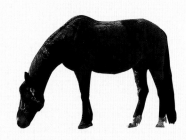

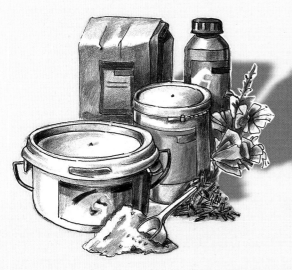

*Because of the huge selection that is available, the feed and supplements market has become confusing.*

Ensure that your horse is receiving a balanced diet, with sufficient minerals and vitamins. If in doubt, seek advice from a qualified nutritionist or contact one of the multitude of help-lines offered by feed companies and consult your vet on the state of your horse's metabolism on a regular basis. It is also sensible, in the case of recurring mud fever, to have a blood count done. Remember also that different feed constituents interact with one another. If you – well-meaningly – give a daily feed of bran mash, a deficiency can arise even with sufficient complete amounts of minerals and trace elements, as individually they will only partly be absorbed. A body may absorb substance A and substance B when they are taken together, but if taken alone substance A may simply be excreted. Other substances are taken up in the same way, a body thus absorbing mineral C or D. Many vitamins can only be metabolised when taken with an amount of fat.

Horse feed should fundamentally always consist of a good source of forage. In the summer this tends to be grass for the majority of horses. As an animal formerly from the Steppes of Central Asia, horses are better off with meagre pasture that has many different plant species, than with a too-rich over-abundance of spring grass.

In winter, sufficient forage also needs to be fed. This will be dried or silaged grass which through this process will have lost much of its goodness. If forage alone is eaten all year round, then an imbalance or deficiency of vitamins and minerals will arise which should be put right through supplementation of feed. Ideally supplementary feed such as course mixes should be given after feeding forage (hay or haylage), so that the stomach is better prepared to metabolise the ingredients. More important than the overall amounts of indi-

## Correct feeding

Equine nutrition and feeding is a highly complex theme and as yet not everything is fully understood. It is certain that a lack of vitamins, minerals or trace elements can work against the natural functioning of the skin. As excess can also unfortunately be harmful, the needs of each horse needs to be calculated individually. Some feeding stuffs visibly work to improve skin, hooves and hair as well as the skin's metabolism.

An over-supply of easily digestible carbohydrates, as often happens in spring on new pasture, appears to increase the chances of feed-induced mud fever occurring.

Metabolic acidosis which can arise through mistakes in feeding is also supposed to increase the chances of mud fever.

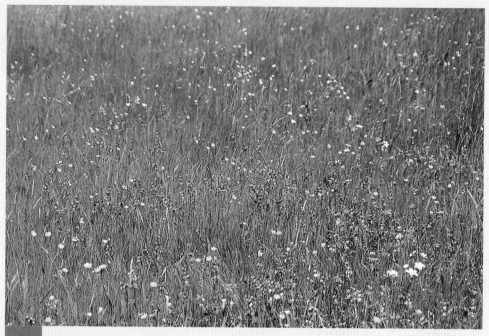

*This pasture looks delicious, but being so lush and with so many buttercups it isn't ideal for horses. Photo: A. Schmelzer*

vidual minerals is the quantities in relation to each other and their availability to the horse. Keep in mind that even when feeding carrots or beetroot in winter, a vitamin deficiency can still occur.

Take care that only the deficiencies and imbalances that exist are rectified. By arguing that, if a small amount helps, then a great deal helps a lot, and feeding too many concentrates, you can actually create new imbalances.

For the general health of the skin various fats and B-Group vitamins are particularly good. Thus feeding sunflower oil, linseed oil or boiled linseed itself can lead to a shiny coat and improved metabolism. Similarly one of the wonders of the feed-store is yeast. Half a cube of yeast a day visibly improves both skin and hooves. But enough of that – this isn't a nutritional guide. Seek advice, ask around and be very sceptical about any feed supplement that promises to cure anything. Good nutrition is the foremost prerequisite for self-healing. Feed is however no medicine!

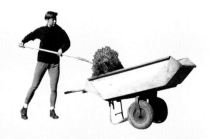

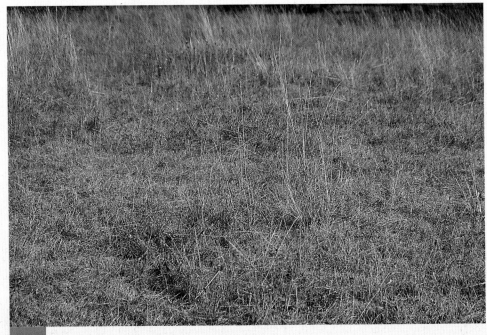

*Slightly sparser pasture is better suited to horses.*
*Photo: A. Schmelzer*

## Mud fever as a warning signal

All eczemas, including mud fever, can also be a sign of some inner illness or imbalance. Liver and kidney disease is always accompanied by detoxification problems that have an effect on the metabolism of the skin. Circulatory problems resulting from illness, hoof problems or lack of exercise also prove harmful to the health of the skin around the pastern.

Infestations of parasites can greatly weaken horses and increase the chances of mud fever setting in. All allergies influence other reactions in the immune system.

Complementary/natural healing methods work on the basis that eczema around the pastern arises when there are problems with the suprarenal glands. Accordingly there could be a connection to the worsening of mud fever under stressful circumstances.

Always keep in mind the health and well-being of the entire horse, even when the immediate problem appears to be limited to the bottom twenty centimetres.

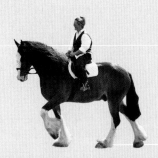

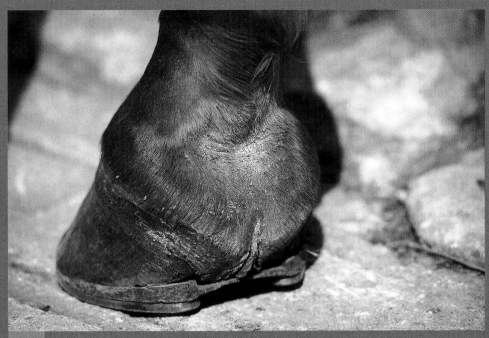

*The skin here looks lightly swollen and feels warm to the touch.*
*Photo: C. Slawik*

# Symptoms of mud fever

*Here you can clearly see the effects of mud fever caused by moisture.*

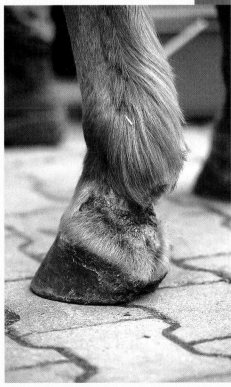

At first a slight reddening of the skin will appear. If you feel the area you will notice some warmth, a light swelling and some pain.

Following this, small nodules and blisters will appear and may burst. The skin is damaged. Small cracks will form that exude serum. On these wounds greasy or crusty scabs will form. It makes a difference in the treatment whether you are dealing with a dry or moist case of mud fever or cracked heel.

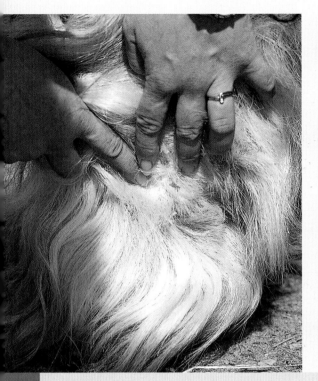

Dry scabs can be hidden under long hair.
Photo: C. Slawik

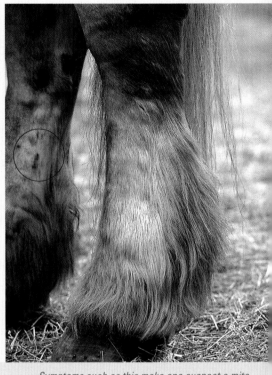

Symptoms such as this make one suspect a mite infestation.

The open wounds can be invaded by various bacteria. Depending on which bacteria are involved the secretions will be greenish, pus-like or rotten-smelling. On the wound a layer will form consisting of serum, dirt, shed skin and hair tissue. This coating offers a perfect breeding ground for a wide variety of germs. In addition it completely blocks the ability of the skin to breathe in the affected area. In some cases fungal infections may also set in, especially where mud fever is treated by frequent washing and antibiotic creams are used.

Thanks to the secretions and at the beginning of the healing process the wound will become itchy. In the case of an attack of cho-

rioptic mange mites this itching is immediate and can affect the whole of the cannon bone. Affected horses may chew at the itchy spots, stamp their feet and scratch themselves on anything available. It can be that a horse plagued by mites will constantly lose its shoes because it is forever scratching its foot on the drinking trough.

If this vicious circle isn't broken, the horse's body will defend itself in its own way. Ideally in the case of a happy, healthy horse kept in good conditions this is successful. The immune system is able to recognise germs and fight them effectively, thus in effect healing itself. This is what we should be striving for. This is

## Clinical stages of mud fever

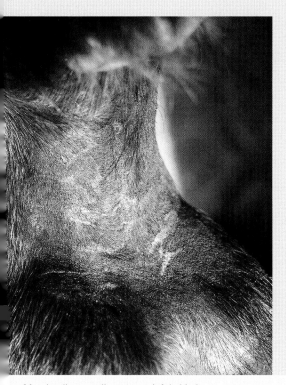

*After healing, small scars are left behind in the pastern. Photo: H. Ende*

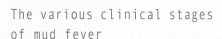

### The various clinical stages of mud fever

**First Stage:** *Dermatitis erythematosa. The skin looks lightly reddened.*
**Second Stage:** *Dermatitis madidans. The skin is slightly swollen and warm*
**Third Stage:** *Dermatitis crustosa: The surface of the skin breaks down and serum starts to leak.*
**Fourth Stage:** *Dermatitis squamosa: The skin swells up and a greasy crust appears on multiple small wounds. Blisters and scabs form and the skin is painful to the touch.*
**Fifth Stage:** *Dermatitis verrukosa. Papillae (small projections) are exposed and growths appear above the usual layer of the skin.*

not possible in all cases, however, because the conditions are not ideal or too much is being asked of the horse's system. In these cases we need to take therapeutic action. The aim is always to re-create the natural function and support self-healing. If the infection advances, then the germs will spread to the deeper tissue layers. The pastern will be painful to the touch and the horse may become lame. Cellulitis and inflammtion of the coronary band may also occur. Where mud fever has broken out the serum will change and the skin will thicken. Effective treatment is now long overdue.

For the treatment and the healing process it is important to recognise at which stage of illness the mud fever is. In stages one and two you can usually manage without washing and disinfecting. Such measures would only irritate and extend the length of time for healing. In stage three it is necessary to get rid of the scabs and clean the area. From the third stage on there will be a hardening of the hypodermis. This is a way of strengthening the layer under the skin, and is accompanied by a loss in ela-

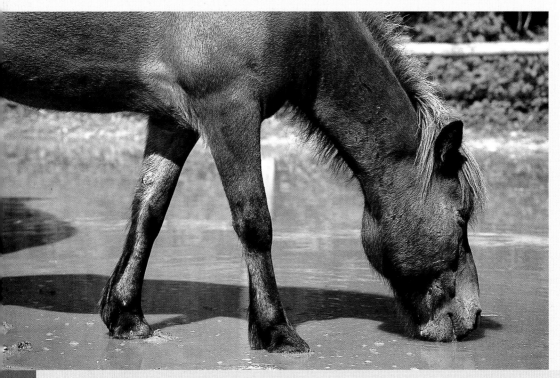

*When a horse is kept in these conditions there is no chance of a case of mud fever healing. Photo: A. Schmelzer.*

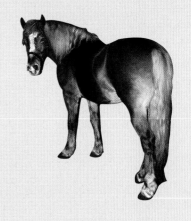

sticity and circulation. Thus the attack becomes chronic and even when the wounds have healed the hypodermis will remain hardened. The next attack of mud fever will occur more easily and will be harder to heal. In the fifth stage only an operation will help, if at all.

The matter is however not as clear as it may seem. There are almost always different clinical stages and degrees of seriousness occurring at the same time on the same leg. You may be familiar with cases where the scabs on the outside are healing well, those on the innermost part seem hardly to change, while those in the middle of the pastern seem to be getting worse.

# What really helps

When treating mud fever, it is of fundamental importance to get rid of the causes. Only then can the treatment be successful.

Take care that your horse has access to somewhere dry for as many hours of the day as possible. Particularly persistent cases, or those horses that have already reached stages four or five, should be stabled full-time. Check what you are feeding them. Remember that you are the one that has to create the conditions under which healing can take place. If lameness, fever or deep wounds accompany the mud fever, then you should always call a vet.

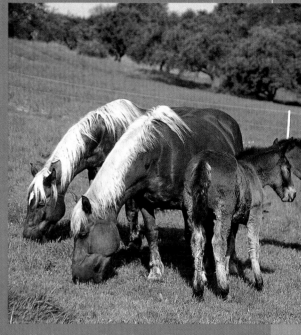

*Mud fever can affect all types. The very stout …*
*Photo: A. Schmelzer*

*… the very big...*

## Orthodox medical treatment

In stages one and two do not wash the wound. For the time being the affected area of the clean and dry leg should be treated with ointment twice a day. A grease-based barrier cream or oil containing zinc oxide, and cod-liver oil or marigold lotions are recommended.

In the case of itching, the use of lotions containing a local anaesthetic is also advised. Such ointments are often not ideal for the renewal of skin but make sense at the beginning of the treatment. You can then break the itching cycle which could lead to the horse rubbing or gnawing its legs, through which new wounds are caused, healing sets in, itching occurs and so on …

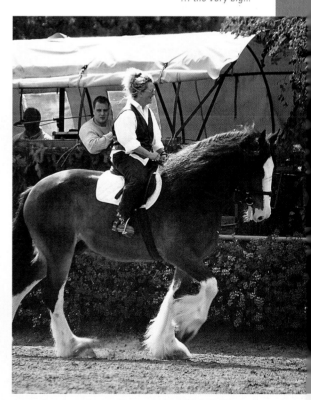

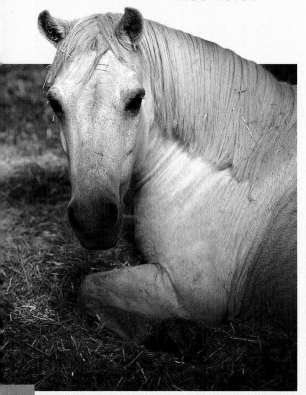

.... and the very small. Photo: C. Slawik

## Treatment with antibiotics

In extreme cases it may be necessary to put the horse on a course of antibiotics. When persistent germs are detected in a wound, the targeted use of antibiotics can prove effective. A prerequisite is that a swab be taken to be bacteriologically examined. Following this, an antibiogram can be completed which should indicate which antibiotics are best suited for use against the infection. There are broad spectrum antibiotics that can be injected or added to feed and which act, as their name implies, on a wide range of germs.

Antibiotics can also be applied in ointments and here too it is sensible to establish beforehand which bacteria are involved and which antibiotic is best suited.

From stage three the affected area should be cleaned with a mild soap once or twice a week. Hibiscrub or another antiseptic or antibacterial solution should be used. After rinsing any soap off it may also be sensible to rinse the area with a three percentage mix of $H_2O_2$ (hydrogen peroxide) or polyvidone iodine (Pevidine solution or similar). Finally a drying powder or an ointment to encourage the regeneration of new skin (epithelisation; often simply described as "healing") should be applied.

Frequently combined ointments are used that contain two types of antibiotic, one to work against fungal infections and a cortisone treatment. Often however this means that there are a number of active ingredients around the wound that are doing nothing.

When using antibiotics, several principles should be observed, regardless of whether they are injected, fed or applied directly to the wound. Antibiotics should only be used when there is no other option. They should be targeted in their use, i.e. ideally after an antibiogram has been done. Antibiotics should always be administered in sufficient doses and for the correct period of time. Always consult your vet, as he/she is the person who should prescribe or administer the medicine. If this advice is not followed then there is the risk that you are just increasing the bacteria's resistance. If the bacteria have been able to build resistance due to under-dosing or

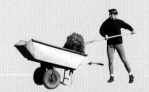

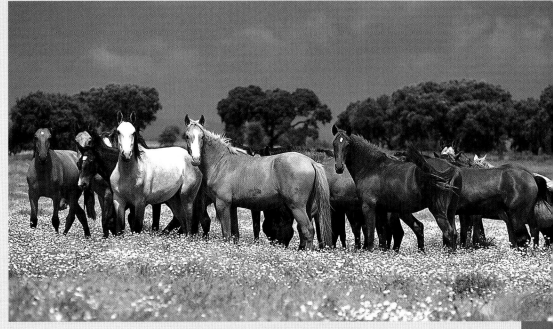

*Every horse is identified and clearly described in its own equine passport. Photo: C. Slawik*

an incomplete course of treatment, then the effectiveness of the antibiotics will be drastically hindered when used correctly.

**Treatment of fungal infections**

If fungal infections also arise as part of the condition there are two other things that you can do for your horse: you can inoculate against infection, and you can treat it with a fungicide. Inoculation against fungal skin infections has been possible for about two years and is a reliable protection against attacks of fungi. In addition this inoculation can impact on the skin's immunity and can thus improve the healing process, if no fungi is involved. Two inoculations, fourteen days apart, are necessary. The

usual precautions should be taken (no stress, and only light work on the day before and after the injection). In rare cases a slight reaction may be noticed after the second treatment. There can be a swelling around the site of the injection, and the horse's temperature may rise slightly. This reaction disappears within a couple of days. Fungicides can in addition be used, dabbed or washed on externally . This type of medicine is available from your vet.

**Treatment of mite infestations**

If mites are involved, then these must also of course be treated. The symptoms of a mite infestation are relatively typical: small scabs will form on the cannon bones (front and back), and these can be scratched off, taking some hair with them. The urge to itch will usually occur. Have a skin and hair sample examined for mites: often these are found very easily. If mites are identified then use a wash or spray treatment against them, following the instructions on the packaging. It may also be possible for your vet to inject a treatment against mites.

Keep in mind that all these treatments are medicines. Their use should be recorded appropriately. According to the appropriate legislation the use of such medicines may have to be documented in your horse's equine passport as well as in an inventory record.

Should your horse not have such a passport (in England at the moment, this is not compulsory) then you can save yourself the bureaucracy and forget about the last paragraph. In those countries where passports have been introduced, not having a current one can be a punishable offence for both the owner and his/her vet. Horse passports are available through breed societies, stud books, national federations (British Equestrian Federation), the British Horse Society and in some cases from veterinarians. Passports are required under most continental European legislation for all horses, whether they compete or not.

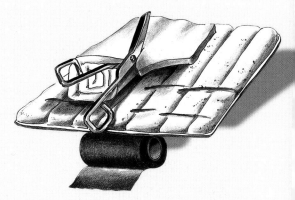

*Here you can see what is required for bandaging the pastern.*

## Bandaging

Back to the subject: In cases of mud fever that have reached stages three and four it may be necessary to bandage the area. These bandages may be for the purpose of disinfection when soaked and applied, or to encourage healing by applying ointment. In all cases the same principle applies: the part of the horse's leg that is to be bandaged must be as clean as possible. You should use a large enough dressing so that the bandages do not stick to the wound, otherwise when you go to change the dressing you will open up the scab again when removing the bandages. This delays the healing process and hurts your horse too.

The next layer of padding should go from the coronet band to the fetlock, but be sure to put enough padding over the area. Over the top, wrap the leg with one of the widely available and usually colourful self-adhesive bandages – neither too firmly, nor too loose. These are relatively expensive but easy to use and they do stay in place. You can of course use other materi-

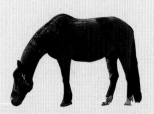

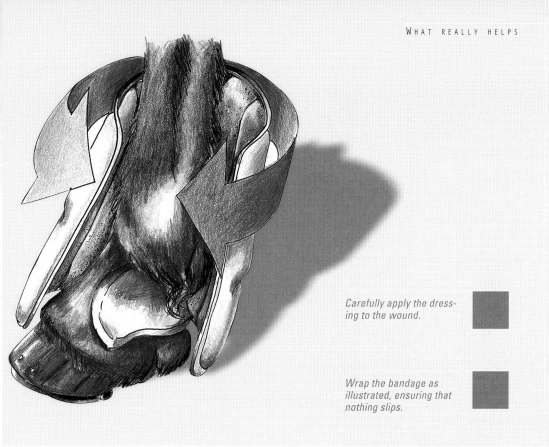

*Carefully apply the dressing to the wound.*

*Wrap the bandage as illustrated, ensuring that nothing slips.*

als so long as they don't stick to the wound and are breathable, but this method is the simplest. It may be necessary to secure the bandage to the hoof with tape, so that it doesn't ride up. Let someone show you how to put on this type of bandage, and practise it on your horse when it is well so that it doesn't matter if you get it right or not. In the long run it means both of you will be more patient.

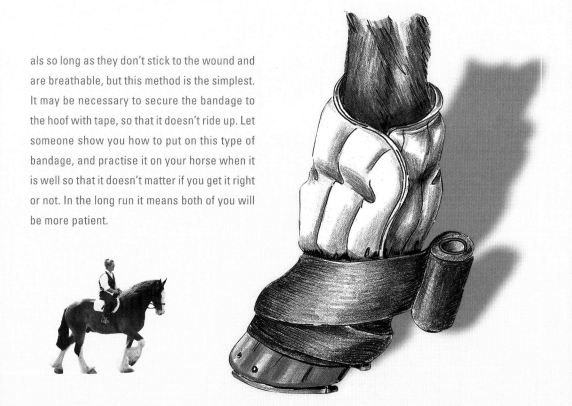

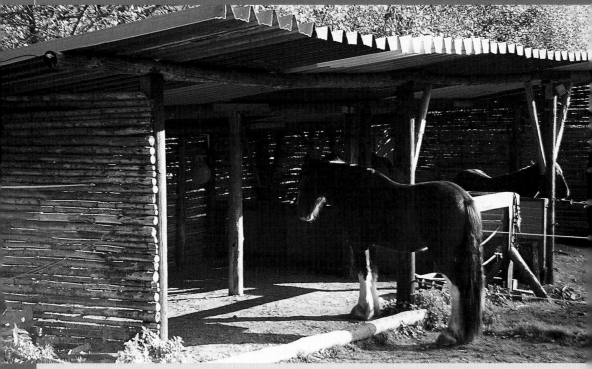

*Don't forget: the way you keep your horse is important. Here it is optimal. Even when it's not summer-time, this shelter will remain dry and accessible. Photo: A. Schmelzer*

# What else can be done?

During the healing process scabs will form. You must watch the wound carefully so that you can treat where treatment is necessary. Good scabs are red and dry and should not be picked off. Yellow crusts and scabs under which it looks greasy should be carefully removed. You may need to soften up these "bad" scabs with soap or ointment, so that their removal doesn't cause pain. Only when the scabs are no longer yellowish or greasy should you try to keep the skin

soft with lotions containing fats. Fat on top of greasy wounds can form an air pocket, and that is to be avoided.

Independent from the clinical stage at which the mud fever is at and in addition to tackling the causes of the attack, there are a number of other things that you can do.

You will improve the chances of a full recovery if you can ensure that your horse has good circulation. This can only be achieved with exercise. It is the hoof that pumps the blood up the leg! As long as your horse is not suffering from great pain and does not have a fever, then it should be led or ridden. In addition it should ideally be turned out for as long as possible so that it can wander at will. At the least it should be taken out of the stable twice a day. Remember that from the moment your horse is stabled, the circulation worsens by the hour until it becomes active again. You can see that for yourself: when you arrive in the morning the horse's legs can be quite thick but after ten minutes of exercise they are much improved. If the legs always swell up so much, the connective tissues can be damaged and pain will be caused.

There is something else that greatly increases circulation, improves the healing process and reduces inflammation. This is the use of soft lasers. Ask whether your vet or complementary therapist possesses such a device. Treatment for only five minutes every second day will greatly enhance the healing process.

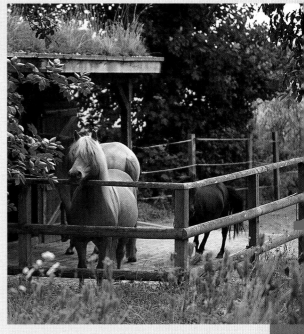

*The ideal turnout – secure fencing with dry shelter. Photo: C. Slawik*

You can assist your horse's recovery by using methods that will systematically impact on the health of the skin and the healing process. This includes good feeding, as already mentioned, and other preventative measures.

Homoeopathic remedies include skin and general health remedies that can be used to help. Silicea and sulphur are often suggested as being effective in treatment. Only someone experienced in homoeopathy, however, will be able to find the appropriate treatment and the correct dosage for your horse and its condition. Homoeopathic treatments are not generic, but rather each treatment needs to be individually diagnosed and implemented.

For the homoeopathic layperson there are a variety of preparations on the market that contain mixtures of various homoeopathic remedies that when used on horses can prove effective. These preparations can be injected, fed or used on acupuncture points. For appropriate advice on which preparations to use, ask your vet or homoeopathist/herbalist.

You can help to increase the ability of your horse's skins to resist attack by having it inoculated against fungal infections (Insol Dermatophyton from Boehringer, see page 23, Treatment of fungal skin disorders).

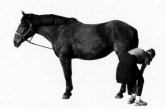

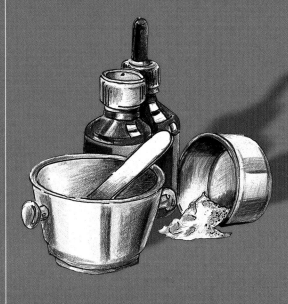

*There are many lotions and creams that can be used.*

# Hints and Tips for the treatment of mud fever

In the next section I will go through some further ideas for treating mud fever that are worth trying. These range from veterinary recommendations, alternative medical therapies and tips from riders, to commercially available remedies. I have not tried out every one of the suggestions, so you will have to see what works best for you and your horse. The list is not exhaustive. There are hundreds of products on the market from the pharmaceutical, cosmetic and equine industries that can be used to treat mud fever/cracked heal. The list is also expressly not a form of endorsement and so if a remedy is included here, it is not meant to imply that it is any better than a product that is not listed. It is purely intended as an overview of a wide selection.

You will frequently see a note advising that attention should be paid to the base used in making the lotion or cream. For one active ingredient there will often be a tincture, an extract, a preparation in an oil-in-water emulsion as well as one in a water-in-oil emulsion and an extract in a fat-based agent. You need to treat the skin but not create an airtight barrier. Moist wounds should dry, dry wounds should stay soft and supple. Always keep that in mind . Neither you nor your vet is the one that is healing – it's your horse that heals. To do this it needs all of its powers of self-healing. You and your vet can help this process along. Tinctures and essential oils may irritate the wound and so should not be used undiluted. Remember too that horses can suffer allergic reactions. Individual horses may be allergic to formaldehyde, tea tree oil or aloe vera. Pay particular attention to whether the chosen product is recommended for use on horses and whether it can be used directly on the wound. When in doubt, consult your vet.

Always observe any advised withdrawal periods. Some preparations contain active ingredients that are so slow to be absorbed that residues may still be detected long after use. Thus even 14 days after their use, a horse can test positive for prohibited substances. If there is a withdrawal period shown, no matter how short, then check with your vet for any potential problems before you compete.

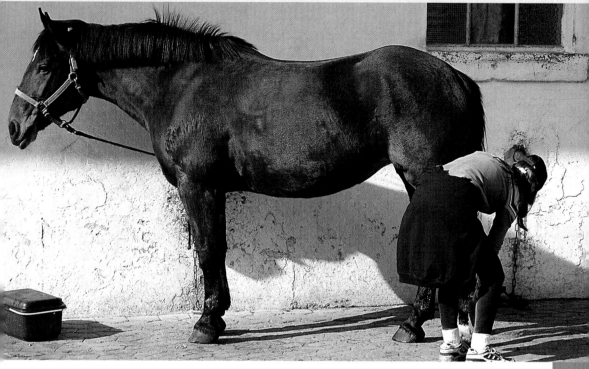

*As part of daily horse care, every horse owner is responsible for prompt and effective treatment. Photo: Schmelzer*

## List of treatments

**Activ Wash:**
An anti-bacterial cleanser which can be used to clean areas prone to mud fever.

**Aloe vera :**
Aloe vera is a plant extract from the plant of the same name that has been used externally in the treatment of wounds for hundreds of years. Aloe vera is often an ingredient in other creams.

**Arnica cream:**
Arnica fosters the healing process. An important factor here is the basis for the cream. Remember that the wound should not be made airtight. Arnica cream should be applied sparingly once a day.

**Baby oil:**
Baby oil can be used to cover and to maintain suppleness of the skin when the healing process is nearly complete.

**Baby powder:**
When the horse is kept in dry conditions baby powder can be sprinkled on moist areas to help dry the wound. Use every second day.

**Broad leaf (wild) garlic paste:**
This is an early-growing plant which has similar properties to (and smells similar to ) garlic. You can make the paste yourself from fresh leaves. Be warned that if you don't use the paste immediately it can sting and be an irritant to the wound.

**Cod-liver – zinc cream:**
This cream has drying properties and fosters the healing process. It can be applied sparsely once a day.

**Dermobion cream:**
This is a medicine that may be used in the initial stages of mud fever when the wounds are causing pain. It contains an antibiotic and local anaesthetic and vitamin A.

**E45 cream:**
E45 cream is intended for human use but it can be effectively used in horses.

**Echinacea cream:**
This contains extracts from the Rudbeckia (black-eyed Susan). This plant can fight germs and improve the natural resistance of the skin. There are also creams available combining echinacea with other plant extracts.

**Fuciderm:**
This is a medicine that is similar to Dermobion. It contains an antibiotic and cortisone and so is suitable for use in painful cases at the beginning of treatment. It smells good and is absorbed quickly.

**Hibiscrub:**
This is an antiseptic solution available from your vet containing chlorexidline, useful in cleaning wounds.

**Marigold cream:**
This encourages the healing process and can be used daily. Watch out what the base of the cream is, to avoid making the wound airtight.

**Mercuchrome:**
This is a solution from human medicine that contains merbromine. It is most suitable as a disinfectant and to dry out wounds.

**Mud fever creams:**
There are many products with various names that fall under this heading. Many vets and companies offer their own special remedies, many of which contain antibiotics.

**Neem cream:**
This preparation comes from an extract of the Neem tree and is a relatively recent development. It works for all forms of eczema and acts in encouraging healing and as a disinfectant.

**Pevidine solution:**
Used for the disinfection and drying out of the wounds.

**Potato starch:**
This can be used to dry out moist wounds in dry conditions when sprinkled on the wound daily.

**Propolis-cream:**
Propolis is extracted from the material used by bees to make hives.

**Sulphur creams:**
A number of sulphur-containing creams exist and can be used successfully in isolation or together with disinfectant creams on moist wounds.

**Sulphur-cod-liver cream:**
Besides healing cod-liver oil, this contains a sulphanomide to fight the bacteria. This should